IN THE CHIA SEEDS WORLD

Grace Rosevear

Contents

Chapter One

INTRODUCTION

The mint plant is related to the chia plant. It produces tiny, flavourless white or dark brown seeds. (Each chia seed has a unique pattern on the shell, ranging from grey to black to tan to off-white.) The nutritional benefits of different seed colours vary slightly. The black seed, for example, provides somewhat more fibre and slightly more protein than the white seed. The anti-oxidant Anthocyanin is also higher in the black seed, which helps reduce free radical damage and indications of premature ageing. The plant pigment anthocyanin is responsible for the colour of dark-colored meals. MySeeds constantly blends black and white chia seeds for best nourishment.

Insects and other pests can't abide the oil that the chia plant produces in its stems and leaves. There's no need to use pesticides when the plant repels bugs safely and naturally.

Chia does not compete with other crops because it thrives in hot, sandy, dry, and poor soil. These factors all contribute to chia being a simple and natural plant to produce.

Chia has no flavour of its own, unlike practically all other foods. It tastes like nothing when it's uncooked. This means you can't dislike it, but it can become monotonous due to the lack of flavour. When you add chia to dishes you already enjoy, it does not dilute or replace the flavours. Instead, it will disperse the flavour or even absorb the flavour of the dish. When you add chia to chocolate pudding, for example, it becomes chocolaty. What about strawberry yoghurt? Then it will have a strawberry flavour.

This overview will help you understand chia and how to apply it to obtain the outcomes you want.

Chia Gel

Chia gel is used as a component throughout the book. When the chia seed is exposed to water or non-acidic liquids, chia gel forms. The soluble fibre on the seed shell's outside hydrates and forms a gelatinous bead around the seed. Chia gel is employed in a variety of ways throughout the book. It can be used to replace butter or oil, to assist tastes blend together, and to add flavour to salad dressings.

The basic ratio "9 to 1" makes chia gel incredibly simple to manufacture. That's 9 parts chia to 1 part water.

1 tablespoon chia seeds, dry

filtered water, 9 teaspoons

Put your chia seeds and water in a resealable container, shake or stir to avoid clumping, and you'll have chia gel in approximately 15 minutes! In a covered container, the gel will last for about a week in the fridge. (If left exposed, it will dry out.) In the kitchen, a spoonful of dry chia goes a long way, so it's also a wonderful bargain.

What is the significance of "filtered water"?

Chia gel isn't designed to taste like anything, however the gelling process can enhance flavours. If there were any unpleasant flavours in the tap water, they might come through in the gel, so use pure water for the best taste.

It's because of this incredible gelling ability that your digestive system treats ordinary water like food. To get to the water, the stomach must first remove the soluble fibre. The gelled seeds will stay in the stomach longer, allowing it to continue transmitting "I'm full" signals to the brain.

Chia can help you achieve a variety of goals, including weight loss by keeping you fuller for longer, giving consistent energy thanks to its high protein level, and offering extra nourishment while reducing fat in your meals. But how can one tiny seed accomplish so much? Take a look at the top ten ways chia can benefit your health.

1.Weight Loss Without Starvation

The Chia Seed is a dream come true for dieters. The tiny, healthful seeds can be flavoured any you wish, and their distinctive gelling action keeps you satisfied for hours. Hunger is a major deterrent to actual weight loss, and you don't want to battle it with jittery, costly medicines. When a chia seed is exposed to water, it develops a gel coating that expands the size and weight of the seed. The gel has 0 calories because it is comprised of water. It's also tough to extract the water from the seed, so it aids your body's perception of fullness without adding calories!

2.Control Blood Sugar

Maintaining healthy blood sugar levels is critical for both health and energy. Blood sugar levels may rise after meals, particularly if you eat high-starchy or sugary foods. This might cause "slumps" throughout your day, making you feel fatigued and drained. You may minimise your risk of type 2 diabetes while also ensuring continuous, consistent energy throughout the day by managing your blood sugar.

What role does the Chia Seed play in this? The seed's gelling activity, as well as its unique combination of soluble and insoluble fibre, work together to slow down the conversion of starches to sugars in your body. If you take chia with a meal, it will aid in the conversion of your meals into constant, stable energy rather than a series of ups and downs that would exhaust you.

3.Aid in the Prevention of Diverticulitis/Diverticulosis

Rich sources of fibre are difficult to come by nowadays, with the profusion of over-processed meals and white flour on the market. Diverticulitis has increased as a result of these quick foods. In this dangerous condition, irregularity is a major component. You need lots of soluble and insoluble fibre in your diet to maintain regularity. The chia seed is here to help if you don't want to eat celery and whole-grain everything—or loads of bran flakes. Soluble fibres are put on each seed to aid in the gelling process. Insoluble fibre protects the seed's outer surface. Because insoluble fibre cannot be broken down or digested by the stomach, the chia seed aids in the smooth passage of food through the digestive system while providing no calories. The seed's soluble fibre and gel coating keep the colon hydrated and allow for simple food transit.

4. Include omega-3 oil in your diet.

Omega-3 oil is commonly referred to as "that good thing in fish." But what if you don't always want to eat fish? What if you're a vegetarian or merely concerned that pollution is contaminating your fish dinner? Chia is the most abundant plant source of this beneficial oil. Chia contains more omega 3 by weight than salmon, and it still tastes delicious! Omega-3 fatty acids are essential for heart and cholesterol health. It's also been touted as a weight-loss aid recently. According to USA Weekend magazine, overweight dieters who included omega 3s in their diet lost two pounds more per month than those who did not.

5.Feel more energy throughout the day

Don't feel like napping in the afternoon? What you eat has a big impact on your energy levels. Chia is one of nature's most complete plant-based protein sources. Protein from foods like peanut butter and some legumes is usually incomplete, which means you must combine it with other foods to obtain the full benefit. Chia, on the other hand, contains a complete protein that will boost your energy levels. Complete protein, vitamins, minerals, and a blood-sugar regulating gel all work together to ensure that you have consistent, never jittery energy.

6.Use less butter while baking

Do you enjoy preparing baked goods at home but despise the amount of butter and oil required? In most recipes, chia gel can replace half of the butter! Because of the chia gel, the food will bake the same and taste the same (or better). Simply divide the amount of butter or oil in half, then fill up the gaps with the equal amount of chia gel. Chia's anti-oxidants can even help keep food fresher for longer. Chia gel can be used to replace butter in cookies, cakes, muffins, pancakes, dessert bars, and more. Which of these recipes will become your new go-to?

7.Incorporate anti-aging antioxidants

Antioxidants are frequently featured in the media due to their numerous health advantages. Antioxidants are abundant in blueberries and some exotic fruits (which aren't constantly in season), but did you know that chia is also strong in them? These beneficial compounds are responsible for the chia seed's long shelf life. They'll keep fresh and ready to eat for over two years at room temperature! And it's all done without the use of any chemicals or preservatives. Other seeds, such as flax or sesame, lack this remarkable potential since they lack the same high anti-oxidant concentration.

Antioxidants protect your body from free radical damage. Free radicals cause problems such as premature skin ageing and tissue inflammation. Stay fresh and healthy by fighting free radical damage with nature's anti-oxidant powerhouse.

8.Reduce food cravings

A lack of minerals or vitamins might cause a hunger for eating. If you're low on calcium, for example, you might feel inclined to consume a lot of cheese and ice cream. This occurs because your body recognises cheese as a calcium source and hasn't been getting enough. What if dairy and whole milk are considered "diet no-nos"? You may always sprinkle chia seeds on your food to increase calcium. Chia provides more calcium per gramme than whole milk. It also contains magnesium and boron, which are important trace minerals for calcium and vitamin absorption. Chia can help you control your cravings by balancing your vitamins and minerals.

9. You can use more flavorful ingredients.

How can a seed with no flavour improve the flavour of things you already enjoy? First, because chia seeds have no flavour of their own, they will never overshadow or disguise the flavour of your food. Second, as the seeds hydrate, the flavour of whatever they were added to is amplified. How about putting them in pudding? Chocolaty! Blend them together in a smoothie? Fruity! Dressings, dips, salsas, sauces, and other condiments are all the same. These two characteristics work together to allow chia seeds to absorb the flavour of whatever they're added to. They disperse your favourite flavours without diluting them.

10. Put money aside

Why should eating less be more expensive? You're probably aware that diet pills are costly, and "box meal plans" can cost up to $500 per month. When you buy "calorie counting packs" or other individual portions in the shop, you're paying more for the preparation and materials that go into each packet. A month's worth of chia costs less than a $1 every day. To obtain your desired outcomes, you can use as much or as little as you like. These basic seeds don't require any special preparations, and they don't even require pesticides to thrive. They're always chemical-free and completely safe. When you're ready to try chia for yourself, all you'll need is a measuring spoon. It doesn't get any easier or more affordable than this.

Want to learn more about how chia can help with specific issues? Interested in learning more about the science behind chia? You can find a variety of intriguing chia seed articles, movies, and more at www.mychiaseeds.com.

"What am I going to do with these chia seeds now that I have them?" you might wonder.

We've put up a list of healthy, flavorful alternatives that you may add to your family's dinners. Chia is ideal for finicky eaters since it can be made to taste like anything. Add fibre and nutrition to your kids' favourite snacks, or try something new! (Wait until you see the adorable chia popsicles!)

Everyone knows that include more fruits and vegetables in your daily diet will help to enhance your immune system and provide you with consistent energy. We want you to be able to do this quickly and easily. We want you to be aware of the ingredients in your food.

There are no chemicals, oil, or high fructose corn syrup in this dish! You can supercharge your body and feel fuller sooner and longer by adding the incredible power of chia.

Cooks like you, not fancy chefs, make up the MySeeds test kitchen. All of the recipes are designed to be simple to create for everyone, using items that can be found in practically any grocery store and only requiring basic cookware. With these simple and nutritious dishes, you may experience the joy of great healthy cuisine and all of its advantages.

Stir-Fry of Chia "Szechwan" in 15 Minutes

DIRECTIONS: Prick the sweet potato peel many times with a fork. Cook for 3 12 minutes on high in the microwave. The middle of the potato should still be solid. Assemble all of the ingredients while the potato is cooking.

Boil the water for the ramen noodles in a 2-quart pot.

Swirl the oil into the hot wok or skillet. Allow it to heat until a few drops of water flicked into the pan sizzle. 1 sweet potato, medium

1 box snow peas, tiny

13 cup bean sprouts or broccoli slaw

fresh spinach, handful

1 teaspoon freshly grated ginger

soy sauce (3 tablespoons)

2 tblsp. olive oil

1 chicken breast (or beef equivalent) sliced into thin strips

1 tbsp chia seed gel

1 teaspoon crushed red pepper

2 ramen noodle bundles (just the noodles you wont need the seasoning packets)

Cook the beef or chicken in a skillet until done (usually just a few minutes). Reduce the stove's temperature.

Add the soy sauce, ginger, red pepper flakes, and chia gel to the pan. Toss to coat. Roll the snow peas in the wok to coat and barely cook them.

Cut the sweet potato into pieces. You want to be able to peel the skin away from the cubes you've sliced and place them in the wok, not cut through it.

Cook the noodles for about 3 minutes, or according to package guidelines, in boiling water.

Top the wok mixture with broccoli slaw or bean sprouts and fresh spinach. Only a tablespoon of the pasta water should be saved after draining the cooked noodles. Roll the noodles about in the wok mixture to coat and wilt the spinach.

Most individuals are aware that seafood is healthy. So it's no surprise that scallops, in addition to their wonderful taste, include thirteen nutrients that can help with cardiovascular health and colon cancer prevention. They're also low in calories! The aromas of this light orange sauce shine through. It serves two people for dinner.

Chapter Two

Stir-fried citrus scallops and vegetables

DIRECTIONS:

Prepare the carrots and spinach beforehand because this meal comes together quickly. Peppers should be thinly sliced.

Begin cooking the pasta in the stock pot according to the package directions.

Combine the orange juice, basil, chia gel, garlic powder, and cornstarch in a small measuring cup. Place aside. 3 oz. spaghetti, uncooked

split in half

12 pound scallops, fresh

2 tbsp. orange juice concentrate + 5 tbsp. filtered water (or 12 cup orange juice)

12 teaspoon cornstarch

12 tbsp basil, dried

a quarter teaspoon of garlic powder

1 tbsp chia seed gel

1 or 2 tablespoons extra virgin olive oil

12 red and orange delicious peppers, each

1 big carrot, cut diagonally

2 cups fresh spinach, torn

Meanwhile, heat the skillet to high heat and drizzle in the olive oil to coat the pan. Adjust the heat a little lower and add the scallops when the oil sizzles when water is flicked into the pan. Brown the scallops for 12 minutes, then turn them and brown for another 12 minutes. They may begin to come apart if you move them around the skillet too much. Scallops should not be overcooked because they will become tough and chewy. Remove the scallops from the pan and place them in a small bowl. When the scallops are left aside, they will continue to cook.

Bring the skillet back up to temperature. Pour the orange juice mixture into the bowl. Toss in the carrots, peppers, spinach, and scallops.

Cook for about 1 minute, or until the spinach wilts. If the sauce becomes too thick, thin it out with a little water. Toss in the drained spaghetti and serve.

Picadillo (pronounced "pic-a-dee-yo") was introduced to us by a Cuban friend. We were sceptical when she said the recipe involved olives and raisins, but it turned out to be tasty and simple. It's not chilli or spaghetti, but it's filling, meaty, and distinctive. It serves two people.

Chapter Three

Chia Picadillo that's almost Cuban

DIRECTIONS:

Cook the ground meat in a large skillet sprayed with cooking spray. Break up the meat and brown it, then drain the fat.

Combine the diced tomatoes, garlic, onion, peppers, raisins, and olives in a large mixing bowl. Stir everything together. Add the cumin, chilli powder, and chia seeds now. Cook for 15 to 20 minutes.

Make the rice according to the package directions while the picadillo is boiling. Add a teaspoon of dried chia to the rice and an additional /s cup water if desired. 12 pound turkey or beef ground meat

1 pound raisins

14 cup olives (green)

12 cup sweet peppers, diced green, red, or yellow (frozen works well)

1 can diced tomatoes, 14 ounces

12 tiny sliced red onion

2 garlic cloves, minced

cumin (1 tablespoon)

1 teaspoon cayenne pepper

1 tablespoon chia seeds, dry

½ cup rice

1 cup of liquid

Curry night is one of our favourites. A vibrant, celebratory lunch results from the passing of all the condiments. Curry is the generic name for a spice mixture found in Asian cuisine. Most curry powder recipes and manufacturers use coriander, turmeric, cumin, nutmeg, and red pepper in their blends. You can adjust the heat level of the sauce to your preference. Curry powder comes in a variety of flavours, so choose one that your family will enjoy. This serves two people for dinner.

Chapter Four

Curr Chia

DIRECTIONS:

Chop the chicken breast, onion, apple, and seasonings into small pieces.

Begin to cook the rice in the cup of water.

In a skillet, cook the chicken pieces and onion until the chicken is no longer pink in the middle. Remove the skillet from the heat and transfer the chicken to the sides. Add the curry powder to the milk and chia gel in the space provided. To evenly spread the powder in the milk, whisk it together. Reduce the heat to low and return the skillet to the stove. Stir in the diced apple and raisins until everything is well combined. Check out the sauce. If desired, increase the amount of curry powder, but keep in mind that the curry powder will bloom and grow hotter. Keep the milk from curdling by keeping the mixture warm.

Examine the rice. Plate the rice and top with the curried chicken mixture after it's done. You can either pass the prepared condiments in tiny bowls at the dinner table or divide them evenly and set on top if you know what your family loves. 1 chicken breast, sliced into small pieces

14 cup onion, diced

1 tablespoon extra virgin olive oil

   cup milk (dairy, almond, coconut, etc.)

12 medium red apples, chopped

14 c. raisins

12 tblsp. curry powder

2 tbsp chia seed gel

½ cup rice

1 cup of liquid

Tomato, cucumber, banana, almonds, and shredded coconut, diced

This hearty meal is ideal for the colder months. Meatless overstuffed potatoes or leftover beef can be cooked. You won't miss the meat if you omit it because it's so filling. Stuffed russet or sweet potatoes are both wonderful. It serves two people.

Chapter Five

Chia Potatoes Overstuffed

DIRECTIONS:

Microwave your potatoes first. Please keep in mind that white baking potatoes take longer to cook than sweet potatoes as you prepare the rest.

Sauté the meat with the minced garlic in a small skillet that has been sprayed with cooking spray. Reduce the heat to medium-low and stir in the ketchup, dry soup mix, vinegar, mustard, chia, and chipotle powder. The sauce will be overly thick, so dilute it with a little water and reduce the heat even further. In the same skillet, coat the remaining vegetables with the sauce.

Warm the mixture until the potatoes are ready. Cut the potatoes lengthwise before serving and split up the centre with a fork to make it simpler to consume. Serve with a serving of the vegetable sauce on top of the potato. 2 baked potatoes, almost the same size, washed and poked many times with a fork

12 cup washed and drained canned red beans

beef, thinly sliced (optional)

1 chopped tomato

1 ear of corn (without kernels) OR

12 cup corn, canned or frozen

a little handful of flat parsley on the left

12 zucchini, peeled and chopped into large bits

1 little sliced sweet pepper

2 garlic cloves, minced

To make the sauce:

12 envelope onion soup mix (dry)

a third of a cup of ketchup

3 tbsp water to thin it out

2 tbsp white vinegar

1 tablespoon mustard (yellow)

chilli powder OR a sprinkle of dried chipotle powder

1 teaspoon chia seeds, dried

Do you need a quick meal? When we're in a hurry, we turn to this pesto. We can create a batch in the mini-chopper for this dinner and then use the leftovers on mozzarella burgers a few days later. It serves two people.

Chapter Six

Pesto with chicken

DIRECTIONS:

To begin, follow the package recommendations for boiling the pasta, ravioli, or tortellini. While the pasta is cooking, combine all of the pesto ingredients in a mini processor and pulse until finely chopped and combined.

Heat the shredded chicken, stock, and sliced olives in a small skillet. Toss in as much pesto as you'll need to "dress" your spaghetti. If necessary, thin with broth. Drain the spaghetti thoroughly. Plate the pasta, top with chicken pesto, and top with tomato slices and a sprinkle of parmesan cheese. spinach chia pesto ingredients

2 big handfuls spinach, fresh

14 cup basil leaves OR

1/8 cup (dry)

basil

2 teaspoons grated parmesan

12 tablespoons extra virgin olive oil

1 big garlic clove

14 cup chicken broth (low salt) (or vegetable broth)

1 teaspoon chia seeds, dried

Dinner's ingredients

12 cup bowtie pasta (dried) OR cheese ravioli/tortellini

1 fully cooked and shredded chicken breast OR shredded leftover rotisserie chicken

a third cup of black olives

1 tomato, thinly sliced into wedges

Adding more broth

This delicious rice will delight your guests. This celebratory dish is somewhat crunchy, slightly sweet, and extremely tasty. It's acceptable for everyone, from omnivores to vegans, as a side dish, and it's also quite simple to prepare. No one will miss the meat with so many delicious flavours. You may easily cook chicken breast medallions to go with the dinner if you want to add more protein. To make the chicken medallions, cut the chicken breast in half lengthwise and then at an angle. Season with black pepper, freshly ground or cracked. Microwave until the inside is no longer pink. Serves four people for dinner.

Rice Has Gone Wild!

FIRST, cook the rice in the veggie broth and water according to the package guidelines, but just until it is slightly undercooked. Remove any seasoning packets that come with the rice. You may prepare the vegetables while the rice is cooking. Cut the tiny carrots into matchsticks and chop the celery. Stir in the thyme and chia seeds once the rice has absorbed the majority of the liquid.

Cut each prune into quarters using kitchen shears or a knife while the rice cools. Remove all stems and coarsely chop the parsley, leaving intact leaves. 1 wild/white rice mix packet

2 celery stalks

12 prunes, pitted

13 cup cranberries, dry

1 handful parsley (flat leaf)

12 carrots, infant

1 cup garbanzo beans or chickpeas

2 tablespoons chia seeds, dry

12 teaspoons thyme powder

1 vegetable broth can (14 oz)

12 cup water, filtered

In a large mixing basin, combine the prunes, cranberries, celery, parsley, and carrot sticks. Drain and rinse the chickpeas before adding them to the bowl.

This can be served hot or cold. Combine the cooled rice with the remaining ingredients in a mixing basin. You're all set to go! Wild rice is a full-grain cereal. It contains more protein and healthful fibre than wheat. B vitamins and magnesium are also found in wild rice. This dish has a high fibre content thanks to the wild rice, dried plums, chia seeds, and garbanzo beans.

This quick Oriental supper pairs sweet and spicy flavours from the tropical pineapple and ginger. The tropical pineapple is sweet and tangy, while the ginger gives the meal a warm flavour.

What's the big deal here? Sweet potatoes! Sweet potatoes have a wonderful texture when they're virtually raw, akin to miniature carrot sticks. The flavour is subtle, unlike a cooked sweet potato. Try it! You'll enjoy it.

This dish serves two to three people.

Chapter Seven

Chia Pineapple Ginger Crunch

DIRECTIONS:

To begin, follow the package guidelines for cooking the rice of your choice. Cut the chicken breast into bite-size chunks while it cooks. Set aside the cubes with the smoked paprika sprinkled on top. Cut the uncooked sweet potato into strips and the white section of the green onion into small rounds to prepare the vegetables. Cut the celery into small pieces.

Cut the cilantro with kitchen shears and grate the fresh ginger root. Spray the cooking surface of a skillet or wok with cooking oil spray and stir-fry the chicken pieces. Add the sweet potato strips, onion, pineapple pieces, and grated ginger once everything is sufficiently cooked. Cook for another 3 minutes.

Combine the lemon juice, cayenne pepper, chia, and honey in a measuring cup. Stir in 1 teaspoon corn starch and 2 teaspoons water. Remove the vegetables from the wok or skillet and pour the mixture in. Slowly stir the mixture until it thickens. When the sauce in the pan has thickened, add the vegetables and chicken and swirl to coat. 1 cubed chicken breast

12 teaspoon paprika (smoked)

3 onions (green) (white portion only)

1 tablespoon ginger root, grated

1 lemon juice tablespoon

12 tablespoons coriander

sunflower seeds, 1 tbsp (per plate)

1 cayenne pepper pinch

1 sweet potato, tiny

2 celery stalks

1 pineapple chunks cup

1 tablespoon chia seeds, dry

½ cup rice

1 teaspoon of honey

12 cup coleslaw dressing (per plate)

corn starch, 1 teaspoon

filtered water, 2 tablespoons

After plating the rice, divide the cooked mixture among the plates. Add the coleslaw mixture on top, followed by the cilantro. Sunflower seeds should be sprinkled on each plate. If sunflower seeds aren't your thing, pine nuts will suffice. Pineapple is both nutritious and delicious! It contains the enzyme bromelian as well as beta-carotene and B vitamins. Bromelian aids protein digestion and maintains the body's alkaline and acidic balance. Pineapple and pineapple juice have anti-inflammatory effects, therefore they may help with a sore throat.

This soup is one of our favourites! It's a hearty dish that can be served cold or hot. Vitamin B6, beta carotene, vitamin D, and magnesium are all abundant in sweet potatoes. It's colourful, tasty, and nutritious! Leave the apple skins on the green apples because the soup will be puréed and you will obtain all of the beneficial fibre. This soup has a slight spiciness to it. This recipe serves four small soup bowls.

Chapter Eight

Sweet Potato Soup with Cream

DIRECTIONS:

In a 3-quart pot, combine all of the ingredients (except the sour cream, black beans, and chia). Stir the spices into the broth to incorporate them. Bring to a boil, then reduce to a low heat and allow it simmer for about 20 minutes.

Allow the "nearly soup" to cool slightly before blending or puréeing. Scoop the bits into the food processor or blender with a ladle or big frying spoon. Make sure not to overpurée the vegetables because the small pieces offer fantastic texture. Combine the sour cream, black beans, and chia seeds in a mixing bowl. We hope you'll have enough for lunch tomorrow! 1 large peeled sweet potato, cut into bits

1 green apple, peeled and sliced

12 medium onions, chopped into slices

chunks

12 cup chicken or veggie

broth

1 teaspoon ginger, grated

12 teaspoon cumin powder

1 teaspoon cayenne pepper

cayenne pepper, 1/8 teaspoon

12 cup sour cream (mild)

1 tablespoon chia seeds, dry

12 cup canned black beans, washed

The aroma of vegetable soup will warm your heart and spirit. Vegetable soup can be nutritious and delicious, especially when you don't have to worry about chemicals in can liners or overcooked or salted food. You know exactly what goes into this soup when you make it! This recipe serves six to eight people. Serve the leftovers for lunch or freeze them for later.

Chapter Nine

Soup with Chia Seeds and Veggies

DIRECTIONS:

Sauté the onion in the olive oil in your large "soup pot." Toss in the tomatoes, cannellini beans, spiced broth, chia seeds, and vinegar. To avoid clumping, stir to include and integrate in the chia seeds. Reduce the heat to a low setting.

Cook the elbows in a second, smaller saucepan according to package directions until slightly underdone. Drain and combine with the soup. Cover and cook for 20 minutes to allow the flavours to meld.

Add the chopped zucchini and spinach leaves just before serving. Gently stir in the spinach until it has wilted. 2 tablespoons extra virgin olive oil

12 diced red onion

2 cans chopped tomatoes (14 oz)

2 c. vegetable stock

oregano, 1 teaspoon

2 tablespoons basil leaves, chopped

paprika, 1 teaspoon

12 teaspoon chilli powder

balsamic vinegar, 2 teaspoons

1 tablespoon chia seeds, dry

1 can washed cannellini beans

34 cup elbow macaroni, cooked

12 peeled and sliced zucchini

1 cup spinach leaves, torn

Chia Fresca, a Mexican cocktail made with fresh lime and chia seeds, inspired this soup. It's hearty with or without the meat because to the sweet potatoes and black beans. It's a one-of-a-kind soup that will liven up your menu. This recipe serves two big soup bowls.

Chapter Ten

Soup with Chia and Lime

DIRECTIONS:

You won't have to slave over a hot burner all day to make this soup. It's a very simple and quick process. To begin, heat the sweet potato in the microwave. It will finish cooking in the soup if you don't cook it all the way through.

Dice the Va jalapeo and cut the tomato into bite-size pieces. Cook the chicken thoroughly in the microwave before cutting into bite-size pieces.

Bring the broth to a low heat in a big pot. In a mixing bowl, combine the jalapeo, cumin, and lime juice. Lastly, add the zest. Remove the tomato from the pot and set it aside. Add the partially cooked yam, chicken cubes, black beans, and baby spinach leaves to the pot, along with the partially cooked yam.

Stir in the dried chia seeds and set aside for 5 minutes to allow the flavours to meld. a quarter of a jalapeo pepper

12 tablespoon cumin

1 medium sweet potato

13 cup dried black beans (rinsed and drained)

1 teaspoon zest of lime (about 1 lime)

1 tablespoon chia seeds, dry

½ tomato

1 chicken breast, boneless and skinless

1 handful fresh baby spinach leaves

1 lime juice tablespoon (about 1 lime)

14 oz broth (chicken or vegetable)

12 tablespoons sour cream (mild) (garnish)

Divide the soup between two large dishes and top with 12 tablespoons light sour cream for a refreshing garnish. This soup should be served warm, not hot. The Advantages of Lightly Cooked Food It has long been recognised that overcooking food depletes nutrition. The "good stuff" in some foods ends up in the cooking water, while it can break down the compounds you required in others. This soup is only cooked for a short time and at a low temperature. Using the microwave to cook the sweet potato and chicken cubes eliminates the need for extensive cooking times and high heat. Beans are heat resistant, and when tomatoes are roasted, they release nutrients. The spinach leaves don't have enough time in the heat to do much more than wilt.

Chapter Eleven

Dressings for Salads

Have you read the amusing article claiming that bottled salad dressing is the thing that lasts the longest in your refrigerator? Two years is the average age! Consider how many preservatives and additives were used to keep those bottles "fresh" for so long. Yikes! It's a little frightening.

Making a fresh batch of dressing as needed would be a preferable option. All of these ingredients are likely to be found in your kitchen on a regular basis. So... keep it fresh! We believe that the dressing should complement rather than mask the flavours of your salad.

You know precisely what goes into these easy, fresh dressings when you create them. There are no artificial colours, preservatives, or tastes. You can't get the same unique flavours from a bottle as you can with fresh fruits and herbs here. The majority of these may be made in about five minutes. You'll also find some delicious salad ideas to go with the dressings. These dressings, on the other hand, should be used on any salad you enjoy serving.

What is your preferred amount of dressing?

For two tossed salads, 4 tablespoons of dressing is generally sufficient. Because of the unique feature of chia gel, hydrated chia works so effectively as a flavour enhancer. It distributes flavour rather than absorbing or diluting it. Because hydrated seeds are mainly water, you're replacing calories and fat with beneficial water without sacrificing any of your favourite flavours! Chia can also be used with store-bought dressings, if you prefer that after learning about these simple homemade dressings.

Why not try this small calorie-saving technique with your favourite store-bought salad dressing?

The secret is to use chia gel in place of 1/3 of the dressing. Dress the salad as usual after mixing everything together. The lower amount of dressing will now cover the same amount of salad and taste the same.

Strong acids (lemon juice, vinegar) and oils (olive oil) will not hydrate chia, but the seeds will cling to the other ingredients.

When you add fruits, nuts, seeds, and veggies to your salads, you add crunch, colour, and a range of macro and micronutrients. Mix things up with a variety of dressings to keep your salads fresh, intriguing, and always in demand.

If you're watching your calories, try this dressing with no additional sugar. Stevia is used to boost the sweetness of the citrus fruits. Its fresh flavour can brighten and complement your favourite greens. Even if you only had a side salad, the chia keeps you feeling full. This dressing contains a full spoonful of dried chia. This dressing will wake up your taste buds and refresh a salad tonight!

Dressing with Creamy Lemon and Lime

DIRECTIONS: Combine the zest, juice, and honey/stevia in a small bowl. Stir in the olive oil. Whisk in the sour cream gradually.

It will keep for about 2 days in the refrigerator. Approximately 3/4 cup dressing 12 cup sour cream (mild)

1 lemon and 1 lime, zest and juice

OR 2 teaspoons honey

12 teaspoon stevia extract

3 tablespoons extra virgin olive oil

a few teaspoons of hot sauce of your choice

pepper, freshly ground

a smidgeon of salt

1 tablespoon chia seeds, dry

With this dressing, make a lovely spinach and strawberry salad! The vibrant greens and reds look delicious. When fresh strawberries are in season, this creates a delicious and unique side salad. When combined with this unique dressing, the baby spinach leaves and strawberries produce a great flavour combination.

Chapter Twelve

Dressing made with apple cider vinegar and olive oil

DIRECTIONS:

Blend all ingredients in a small mixing bowl and whisk to combine. If you leave it for a minute, it will split. For the finest flavour, shake or mix your salad before dressing it. 14 cup extra virgin olive oil

2 tbsp. honey OR

12 teaspoon stevia

apple cider vinegar, 2 tablespoons

1 tablespoon chia seeds, dry

1 teaspoon Worcestershire

1 paprika dash

Lemon and basil go well together, and Dijon mustard adds a little zing. Use olive oil to dress your salad, especially if it contains fat-soluble elements like lycopene, beta carotene, and lutein. These nutrients are best absorbed when consumed with a small amount of healthy fat, such as olive oil.

Chapter Thirteen

Vinaigrette with Lemon

DIRECTIONS:

In a small container, combine the lemon juice, Dijon mustard, and honey. Slowly drizzle in the oil while whisking constantly. Approximately 3/4 cup 3 tablespoons of lemon juice OR 1 lemon

juice of lemon

1 tablespoon mustard (Dijon)

1 tblsp. honey

6 tablespoons extra virgin olive oil

2 tablespoons chia seeds, dry

salt to taste

2 tablespoons fresh basil, clipped

It's delicious with mixed greens, oranges, avocado, kiwi, and/or strawberries. The raspberry's sweet-tart flavour pairs well with other fruits. Fruit salads are nutritious, bright, and enticing.

Chapter Fourteen

Dressing with raspberry vinegar

DIRECTIONS:

In a small mixing dish, whisk together the ingredients.

13 cup plain yoghurt

raspberry vinegar (2 tbsp)

1 tablespoon maple syrup (optional)

honey

1 teaspoon chia seeds, dry

Vinegar of raspberries

If your grocer has a specialised vinegar department, you can buy raspberry vinegar there. However, it may not be available at all times or may be costly. Fortunately, you can create this yourself at home! If you store it in a glass container, it will last longer. Once you've made raspberry vinegar, you'll be shocked at how many diverse uses you can find for it. Make raspberry vinegar as follows: In a small bowl, combine V cup white vinegar and V cup raspberries (fresh or frozen). Overnight, soak the vinegar and fruit. The next day, smash the berries in the vinegar with a spoon to extract as much juice and flavour as possible. Strain the raspberry pulp through a sieve and pour the vinegar into a clean, covered glass jar. It's vital to avoid using plastic around strong things like vinegar since it can leach toxins into your meals. When cooking fresh salads, you'll be amazed how often you grab for your fruited vinegar.

This dressing goes well with fresh spinach and a variety of fruits and vegetables. It won't wind up on the plate or at the bottom of the bowl since it's so thick. Chef salads benefit with the addition of grilled chicken. Sprinkle roasted sunflower seeds on top for added crunch.

Salad Dressing with Strawberry Chia Chef

DIRECTIONS:

Pulse the strawberries and vinegar together in a food processor. Add the pepper and chia seeds once they've been chopped. This dressing is thick and adheres to all of your salad toppings. 1 cup strawberries (fresh or frozen)

1 tablespoon balsamic vinegar

vinegar balsamic

1/8 teaspoon pepper, ground

2 tablespoons chia seeds, dry

Do you enjoy French dressing? Try out this new twist. You won't want bottles of dressing with preservatives and additives lying around your fridge because it's so simple to create. Simply prepare a batch anytime you feel like a salad.

Chapter Fifteen

"French Dressing"

"French Dressing" is a term used to describe a type of dressing.

DIRECTIONS:

In a small mixing bowl, whisk together all of the ingredients to combine, and you're done! Toss in as much black pepper as desired. Many foods, including black pepper, help your body absorb nutrients more efficiently. 14 cup extra virgin olive oil

ketchup (14 cup)

3 tablespoons sugar OR stevia or other sugar alternative

xylitol

white wine vinegar, 3 teaspoons

1 teaspoon powdered garlic

2 tsp Worcestershire sauce a pinch of salt and pepper

1 teaspoon chia seeds, dry

Have you ever tried Lemon Chia Vinaigrette? This velvety Dijon is a must-try. Mustard has a lot of antioxidants and offers a lot of flavour without adding any calories. This flavorful, creamy alternative dressing is loaded with garlic.

Chapter Sixteen

Creamy Yogurt Chia Dijon

Dressing

DIRECTIONS:

Combine the ingredients in a small bowl and let aside for 15 minutes. The garlic will have time to infiltrate the dressing and the chia will have time to assist mix the flavours. This recipe makes about a cup. 12 cup plain low-fat yoghurt

three tablespoons Mustard dijon

lemon juice, 3 teaspoons

1 tablespoon honey OR sugar

1 garlic clove, diced, salt and pepper

2 tablespoons chia seeds, dry

We adore this rich "south of the border" dressing, which may remind you of some of your favourite Mexican eateries. This lighter dressing/sauce can also "liven up" a wrap or sandwich. It's simple to double the ingredients.

Chapter Seventeen

"It's Only a Little Kick" Chia Dressing

(Southwestern)

DIRECTIONS:

Simply combine all of the ingredients in a small bowl and set aside. If you're having a taco salad or preparing edible bowls (see page 109) for a creative presentation, this is a great option. 14 cup plain low-fat yoghurt

14 cup sour cream (low fat)

1 coarsely minced tiny garlic clove

212 tablespoons chilli of your choice

sauce

a squeeze of lemon a pinch of cayenne

1 teaspoon chia seeds, dried

The sharpness of fresh lime is a lovely counterpoint to the sweetness of the dessert. Strawberries and apples go great together, but so are little sliced dates or even grapes. The dressing is neither heavy or heavy, and it always seems light and fresh.

Chapter Eighteen

Desserts

Do you enjoy sweets? Do you wish there were some that were better for you? Try these delicious chia treats. You won't want to go back to the preservative-filled, dried-up box cookies on the shelf after making a few fresh-baked, uncomplicated cookies. Hopefully, these examples show how real fruit (rather than "fruit-flavored replacements") can enhance the flavour of your desserts.

Chia is utilised in two ways in these desserts:

Cut the fat—When half the butter, oil, or shortening in a dish is replaced with chia gel, the result is a dessert with half the fat of the "normal version." However, as you'll see, it bakes, looks, and tastes exactly like the full-fat version.

Add moisture—Reducing fat content can result in dry sweets. This isn't a problem because the chia gel adds moisture. You'll see what we mean when you try the smooth, delectable crumb in dishes like the Easiest Carrot Cake (page 171)

Chia is a great way to make dessert time healthy. But that doesn't give you carte blanche. You can't have dessert if you don't have any fat or sugar. That's where chia's ability to "full you up quickly" comes in useful. A little goes a long way in these deserts.

Ingredients for dessert:

These desserts don't contain any uncommon, pricey flours or specialised store items.

These recipes are simple enough for anyone to prepare. If you wish to use carob chips instead of chocolate chips, that's fine, but it's not required.

Love the classic snickerdoodle's fluffy, puffy texture? There are three alternative ways to produce these now! They're great with cinnamon sugar, but you can also try cinnamon mini-chips and cinnamon pecans. Even though they're half the fat, these snickerdoodles have the airy, fluffy texture you adore and fill the house with cinnamon fragrances while they bake. This recipe makes around fifty cookies.

Chapter Nineteen

Snickerdoodles with Chia

DIRECTIONS:

Combine the flour, salt, and baking powder in a mixing bowl. To blend, whisk everything together thoroughly. Cream the sugar and butter together in a large mixing basin using an electric mixer. When finished, it should seem pale and gritty. Add the eggs next, mixing thoroughly after each addition. After that, stir in the apple sauce. Finally, by hand, incorporate the chia gel.

Slowly incorporate the flour mixture into the butter mixture. The dough will thicken. If the dough is too sticky to roll, put it in the fridge for 15 minutes.

You can create three different types of cookies or stick to one topping for the entire batch. In a small bowl, combine 1 tablespoon cinnamon and 2 teaspoons sugar, then scoop 1 tablespoon dough into the mixture. To coat the dough ball in cinnamon-sugar, gently shake or roll it. Ingredients (Dry)

334 cup flour

2 tblsp. baking powder

1 pound of sugar

12 teaspoon sodium chloride

1 tablespoon cinnamon powder

Ingredients in liquid

9 tablespoons margarine or butter

2 eggs

12 cup sugar-free

sauce with apples

7 tablespoons chia seeds, gelled

Ingredients to Consider

chocolate chips, mini

pecans, chopped

The cinnamon-sugar on the outside of these cookies complements the pecans well. To help pecans stick to the dough, chop them into little pieces. Place the pieces in a basin with cinnamon and sugar.

Add small chocolate chips to your cinnamon-sugar bowl to produce the chocolate variation. Only micro chips will work because larger chips will get stuck in the cookie dough as it is swirled around in the mixing. The flavour combination of cinnamon and chocolate is fantastic!

Place each cookie on buttered baking trays once it has been coated. Preheat oven to 350°F and bake for 13 minutes. The edges should be gently browned when done, and the cookie tops should be firm.

The cinnamon-sugar on the outside of these cookies complements the pecans well. To help pecans stick to the dough, chop them into little pieces. Place the pieces in a basin with cinnamon and sugar.

Add small chocolate chips to your cinnamon-sugar bowl to produce the chocolate variation. Only micro chips will work because larger chips will get stuck in the cookie dough as it is swirled around in the mixing. The flavour combination of cinnamon and chocolate is fantastic!

Place each cookie on buttered baking trays once it has been coated. Preheat oven to 350°F and bake for 13 minutes. The edges should be gently browned when done, and the cookie tops should be firm.

No shortening in the pie crust? A pie that is virtually healthy? Also gluten-free? That would be a real delight. You will be delighted if you try this dish. Are you in a hurry? This method can also be used with a store-bought crust (even the chocolate coating part of the recipe). Use white chips instead of chocolate to make a white chocolate coating. The delicious chocolate covering on the crust keeps the crust firm and never mushy. This produces one eight-inch-diameter pie.

DIRECTIONS: In a mixing dish, combine the above ingredients and pack down so that the juice from the grated apple pervades the oats. Allow 10 minutes for the mixture to rest. If the apple isn't particularly juicy, add 1 teaspoon of water to help the ingredients stick together and form the crust.

Preheat oven to 375 degrees Fahrenheit. Using cooking spray, coat an eight-inch pie tin. Press the oat crust into the pan and up the sides evenly. Melt the chocolate chips while the crust is cooking, around 15 minutes. Melt the chips in a microwave-safe measuring cup on high for 33 seconds, mix, and continue melting for 22 seconds. Stir and set aside until the pie is cool. Allow the crust to cool while you prepare the filling.

Whip the cream in a large mixing basin with an electric mixer until it is firm. Place this in the refrigerator. Combine the 2 yoghurt cups and the dry vanilla pudding in a mixing basin. Combine everything in the mixer. Don't worry if the mixture becomes thick and pasty; the next ingredients will loosen it up.

Next, add the tablespoon of milk and the tablespoon of sugar to the mixer. Make the pie crust as follows:

1 peeled tiny green apple

and grated, which equals

½ cup

114 rolled cups

salt and oats

1 teaspoon sugar (brown)

1 tablespoon oil (vegetable)

1 tbsp chia seed gel

12 CUP COOKIE CHIPS

Filling ingredients:

12 cup thawed frozen raspberries

2 small glasses raspberry juice (6 oz)

yoghurt with low fat

1 vanilla instant pudding box

2 tbsp chia seed gel

1 tablespoon almond milk OR rice milk

12 cup heavy cream, whipped

chia gel. To prepare raspberry juice and purée, smash 12 cup of raspberries with a fork in a small bowl. Stir it into the pudding mixture with a spoon. You can add another tablespoon of milk if the mixture is still very pasty or appears dry. Fold in the whipped cream and entire berries with care.

Spread the chocolate evenly over the crust with the back of a spoon.

The pie shell should now be cold enough to handle. To coat the crust, evenly spread the melted chocolate. Working with the back of a spoon, be careful not to pull crumbs from the crust. This creates a "moisture barrier," preventing the crust from becoming soggy.

Place the entire chocolate-covered crust in the freezer for about 10 minutes after coating. This will help the chocolate layer to set.

Fill the pie crust with the raspberry filling and place it in the freezer. In around 4 hours, it should be solid. The pie should be placed out on the kitchen counter to "warm up" a little before serving so that it may be sliced easily. Why not use fat-free or low-fat whipped cream instead? High fructose corn syrup, hydrogenated vegetable oils, corn syrup, and preservatives are all common ingredients. Trans-fats in hydrogenated vegetable oils can elevate harmful cholesterol levels. When you look at a package of whipped topping, you'll see at least 5 and up to 18 ingredients. There is only one ingredient in whipped cream (that you whip yourself).

What is a chiffon cake, exactly? The lightness of a "angel food" cake is combined with the richness of a butter-based cake. Fantastic! It's a "traditional" cake that you won't find in restaurants or cookbooks. It's also not available in a box mix. Choose this Marbleized Chiffon to wow your guests with a delectable dessert they've probably never had before.

The cake "rises" atop egg whites, giving you protein without the calories, so you'll need an angel food cake pan. Don't worry if it appears more difficult than it is; this cake is well worth the effort.

Chapter Twenty

Cake with Marbleized Chiffon

DIRECTIONS:

In a medium mixing bowl, sift together the flour, baking powder, salt, and sugar. To place the egg yolks, make a bowl-shaped depression in the flour.

Separate the eggs next. If the yolk cracks and penetrates the white, the whites will not beat to a "stiff consistency" later. Fill a large non-plastic dish halfway with each white. (Because the whites will whip up to a high temperature, the bowl should be larger than usual.)

Microwave Va cup water for about 30 seconds in a 1 cup measuring cup. 2 tablespoons sugar and 1 unsweetened chocolate square With a spoon, break up the chocolate and mix to blend. While you move on to the next stage, let it settle and melt together.

Preheat oven to 325 degrees Fahrenheit. Remove the angel food pan from the oven. Important: Don't oil or spray anything!

Return to the large bowl of egg whites after that. Add the cream of tartar (12 teaspoon). Beat on high with an electric mixer until stiff peaks form. With a spatula, you should be able to cut through them. 214 cup cake flour, sifted

12 pound sugar

a third teaspoon of baking powder

1 tblsp. salt

14 cup oil (vegetable)

7 distinct eggs

34 cup ice water

14 cup chia seed gel

1 teaspoon vanilla extract

12 teaspoon tartar sauce

For the batter, chocolate

14 cup of water

2 teaspoons of sugar

1 square (1 ounce) unsweetened bakers chocolate

filtered water, 14 cup

2 teaspoons of sugar

corn syrup (two teaspoons)

14 cup cocoa powder, unsweetened

14 cup chocolate chips, semi-sweet

Return to the basin with the flour and egg yolks. Add the vanilla, 34 cup cold water, and the vegetable oil. Beat until smooth with an electric mixer.

Gently fold the stiff egg whites into the flour/egg yolk batter as it slowly pours over them. Bring the spatula up and over the egg whites from the bottom. You want to maintain all of the air in the egg whites that you whipped in. Fold the batter until it is homogeneous.

Always use a serrated knife and a sawing motion to cut an angel food cake.

Fruits like strawberries or raspberries can be served alongside this light, tasty cake. Do you want anything really decadent? Here's how to make a quick chocolate sauce:

Microwave for 30 seconds with all ingredients in a microwave-safe measuring cup. Stir everything together. You're done! Microwave for another 20 seconds or less. If you leave it out on the counter to cool, it will solidify a little. Simply re-heat in the microwave to re-liquefy.

To keep the chocolate liquid, most ganaches contain heavy cream, butter, or oil. This recipe has a deep chocolate taste and only utilises a minimal quantity of oil in the chips. Use this not only with this cake, but anytime else you want a chocolate drizzle.

Remove 13 cup of the batter and stir in the already melted and chilled chocolate. To make the chocolate batter for marbleizing, fold again to mix.

Ready? Half of the light batter should be poured into the 10" angel food tube pan. Half of the chocolate batter is dolloped on top. Pour the remaining light batter over the top. Finally, make more dollops with the remaining chocolate batter. To generate the marble look, gently swirl the batters using a knife or narrow spatula. Leave distinct light and dark batter sections.

Preheat oven to 325°F and bake for 65 minutes. When lightly pushed with a finger, the cake will spring back.

Invert the cake into the pan and set aside to cool. Most tube pans have small "feet" on which to invert the cake. Gently slide a knife along the edge of the cake as well as the middle tube to remove it. To release the cake, pull up on the central tube. To loosen the cake from the bottom of the pan, carefully run the knife under it. Voila! Your dessert! What's the difference between all-purpose flour and cake flour? The amount of protein. There are 11 percent in all-purpose flour and 6 percent in cake flour. A lighter cake is made with less gluten/protein. This cake requires cake flour, and replacing is not advised.

Chewy and crunchy chocolate chip cookies are the two most common textures. This recipe makes the chewiest, most delectable chocolate chippers you've ever tasted. Stay clear if you like crunchy cookies; these bake up fluffy, light, and never oily. Large, gooey chocolate chips abound in these soft, moist cookies. They're delicious right out of the oven and keep well in airtight containers. They should be refrigerated after a few days to avoid mould because they are moist and rich-tasting with no preservatives. The number of cookies you receive is determined on the size you select from the list on page 165.

Chapter Twenty-one

Chia Chocolate Chip Cookies

DIRECTIONS:

Preheat the oven to 325°F and oil your cookie sheets first. Blend the melted butter with both sugars until smooth. The vanilla, applesauce, whole egg, and egg yolk are then added. Stir again until everything is well blended. Last but not least, whisk in your chia gel. Combine the remaining dry ingredients in a separate bowl, excluding the chocolate chips (flour, baking soda, salt). With a wooden spoon, slowly incorporate the dry ingredients into the wet ingredients. Only stir until everything is well blended. Add the 2 cups chocolate chips last.
Ingredients (Dry)

flour (two cups)

12 tablespoons baking soda

12 teaspoon sodium chloride

14 cup granulated sugar

1 pound of brown sugar

2 cups chocolate chips, semi-sweet

Ingredients in liquid

8 tablespoons butter, melted

4 tbsp chia seed gel

a quarter cup of apple sauce (unsweetened)

1 teaspoon vanilla extract

1 complete egg

only 1 egg yolk

Note that most cookie recipes only make a specific size of cookie. If you try to create the cookies at a size that isn't specified in the recipe, you'll end up with undercooked cookies with burned edges, or overdone cookies despite the baking time. These cookies can be created in three different sizes. You can use giant chocolate chips or chocolate chunks if you're creating large or medium-sized cookies. Regular-size chocolate chips work well when baking medium or small cookies.

Use 14 cup scoops of batter for enormous cookies and bake for 15 minutes. Use 112 tablespoon scoops of batter for medium cookies and bake for 12 minutes. Use 112 teaspoon scoops of batter for smaller cookies and bake for around 10 minutes.

The cookies will be golden brown when done baking. Although the edges will be somewhat toasted, the centres will remain soft and puffy. Take care not to overcook.

Our friend Florence is a fruit crisp enthusiast and is frequently one of our taste testers. This chia fruit crisp is one of her all-time faves, according to her. Let's see whether it turns into one of yours as well. You may make this crisp with any seasonal fruit or buy it frozen at your local supermarket. The spices in the topping complement the fruit flavours and help keep the crisp topping crispy. The apples give this bright, uncomplicated dessert a lovely texture. This yields an 8 by 8 crisp, which is normally divided into nine squares.

Chapter Twenty-two

Crispy Chia Triple Fruit

DIRECTIONS:

Preheat oven to 400 degrees Fahrenheit. Using cooking spray, coat an 8 × 8 baking dish.

Stir together the brown sugar, cornstarch, and orange juice in a large pot until smooth. Cook, stirring occasionally, until the sauce has thickened. Combine the cinnamon, nutmeg, chia, lemon juice, and a pinch of ground cloves in a mixing bowl. Remove from the heat and coat the fruit in the sauce. Fill the baking dish halfway with the fruit mixture.

Combine the flour and spices in a small bowl. Cut in the butter until coarse crumbs are formed. Mix in the granola and dry oats. Stir everything together. Over the fruit mixture, sprinkle.

Bake for about 25 minutes, or until the topping is golden brown. Serve with a friendly grin. 12 cup peaches, sliced (with or without peels)

12 cup blueberries, fresh or frozen

2–3 sliced tiny green apples

1 lemon juice tablespoon

a quarter cup of orange juice

Crisp topping ingredients:

granola (14 cup)

14 cup oats (quick cooking)

14 cup of flour

4 tbsp. chilled butter, sliced into tiny pieces

a pinch of cinnamon

nutmeg (12 teaspoon)

Strawberry fans, rejoice! This is the cake you've been looking for! This cake offers a blast of actual strawberry flavour in every mouthful, thanks to two cups of strawberry purée. This cake can be made with fresh or frozen berries and is suitable for any season. When you drizzle sweet-tart strawberry dripping over a warm slice of this extremely berry bunt cake, you don't need buttery icing. A typical 10/4 inch bunt cake is made with this recipe. This cake will be light tan in colour when baked, with pink strawberry bits scattered throughout like confetti. It won't be brilliant pink until food dye is used.

Chapter Twenty-three

Super Strawberry Chia Cake

DIRECTIONS:

Sift together the cake flour, baking powder, salt, and sugar in a medium mixing basin. Then puree 112 cups strawberries. You can use a food processor, a small chopper, or a blender. The number of berries required is determined by the size of the berries. After sifting the dry ingredients, crack all four eggs into a small basin and whisk vigorously to combine. Return the eggs to the whisk and add the chia gel and vegetable oil.

Pour in the wet ingredients first, followed by the strawberry purée. Mix with a wooden spoon until everything is well combined. Strawberry chunks will be visible in the cake mixture, which will be fairly thick.

Spray your bundt pan with non-stick cooking oil spray and set aside. Depending on the pan, you may want to coat the inside with flour as well to ensure that the cake comes out easily. Pour the batter into a bundt pan and bake for 45 minutes at 325 degrees. When the cake is done, it should spring back when softly pressed. Ingredients (Dry)

3 cups cake flour, unbleached

a third teaspoon of baking powder

12 teaspoon sodium chloride

134 cup sugar, white

Ingredients in liquid

4 eggs

12 cup oil (vegetable)

14 cup chia seed gel

12 cup pure strawberry

Ingredients to Drizzle

12 cup pure strawberry

1 teaspoon of sugar OR

14 teaspoon stevia extract

Purée roughly 12 cup of strawberries to produce the strawberry drizzle. Add the 1 tablespoon of sugar and pulse to blend once they're chopped. While the cake bakes, set this aside because the sugar will remove part of the purée's liquid. Slice the cake into slices and drizzle with the mixture to serve. Why is cake flour used? The protein content of cake flour is lower than normal flour. It is because of this property that a cake remains light and fluffy. This recipe calls for cake flour because the enormous amount of berries would otherwise result in a heavy cake.

When you realise how simple this recipe is, you'll never go back to store-bought carrot cakes. As it bakes, the warm spices fill the house with a delightful aroma. It's more moist and flavorful than anything from a box mix or off the store because of the unusual components. Real, fresh fruits and veggies are the best! You won't even need heavy cream cheese frosting because the cake is sweet enough. This recipe yields a 13 x 9-inch cake.

DIRECTIONS FOR THE EASIEST Chia Carrot Cake:

Preheat the oven to 375 degrees and grease a 9 x 11 or 13 x 9 baking dish.

Combine the flour, spices, and baking soda in a medium mixing basin.

With an electric mixer, whisk the purée, carrots, sugar, crushed pineapple, eggs, and vanilla in a second large mixing basin until well combined. Hand-stir in the chia gel with a spoon.

Combine the wet and dry ingredients in a medium mixing basin. Stir everything together. Bake for 30–35 minutes, or until a toothpick comes out clean, after spreading the batter evenly in the pan.

Allow to cool completely on a wire rack before cutting into squares.

Allow to cool completely on a wire rack before cutting into squares.

2 cups flour (all-purpose)

sugar (34 cup)

2 tablespoons cinnamon powder

18 teaspoon cloves, ground

112 tsp baking soda

salt to taste

Ingredients in liquid

12 cup pineapple juice (crushed)

a quarter cup of prune purée

4 medium grated carrots (about 4 cups)

2 eggs

3 tbsp chia seed gel 2 tblsp vanilla extract Please don't be alarmed, but we read an article about prune purée about a zillion years ago and remembered that it adds richness and sweetness to a recipe without adding the actual flavour of prunes. To achieve the same fantastic taste and texture, use prune purée instead of refined sugar and oil. Place 34 cup prunes and 14 cup extremely hot water in your food processor/mini chopper to make prune purée. Pulse until the ingredients are finely chopped into a paste. Add a bit more water if necessary to keep the paste from becoming too thick. More purée? It will last around two weeks in the fridge if kept in an airtight container.

Without the wheat, they are a simple delight! Despite the lack of flour, these cookies bake up crisp on the exterior and chewy on the inside. Because they're made with all-natural, unsweetened peanut butter, they're bursting with peanut butter flavour. When a cookie becomes overly sweet, it might mask the flavour of the other ingredients, leaving only the sweetness. By using unsweetened peanut butter, this is easily prevented. Do you want even more nuttiness? You can use whole peanuts or peanut butter chips in this recipe. Don't skip the nutmeg, even if it's only a pinch. It's quite mild, but it gives the peanut flavour a nice richness. This recipe makes around forty cookies.

Chapter Twenty-four

Peanut Butter Cookies without Gluten

DIRECTIONS:

You can make these cookies while the oven is preheating to 350 degrees.

To begin, cream the butter and both sugars with an electric mixer until a light, grainy texture forms. Then, one by one, add the eggs, mixing after each addition. Add the vanilla, nutmeg, and baking soda after that. Hand-mix in the chia seeds. Stir in the peanut butter with a large spoon until everything is thoroughly mixed.

Add the oats last, one cup at a time, along with your preferred chips (or peanuts). Once you've added all of the oats, the batter will become very thick and difficult to stir. A cookie scoop or measuring spoon can then be used to scoop it onto greased cookie sheets. Small cookies, about 2 tablespoons apiece, are ideal. Because they don't spread much, they can be placed near together on the sheet. Ingredients (Dry)

3 cups oats (quick cook)

12 cup sugar, white

12 cup sugar (brown)

112 tsp baking soda

1 tsp. nutmeg

12 tablespoons salt

1 chocolate chip cup (or peanut butter chips)

Ingredients in liquid

2 eggs

1 teaspoon vanilla extract

2 tbsp. melted butter (softened)

1 cup unsweetened natural peanut butter

chia seed gel (two teaspoons)

Cook for approximately 10 minutes. (Take care not to overcook! These are prone to drying out.) When the edges and bottoms of the cookies are just browned, they are ready. These will keep for approximately a week in an airtight container.

The cake will be moist and soft without being overly sweet because it is made using brown sugar. Fresh orange zest gives a pop of flavour without changing the texture of the dish. A small slice of this refined and rich cake can fulfil a chocolate hunger. This recipe yields a 9-inch round cake.

Although this cake does not require frosting, it is delicious when served with a vivid orange sauce (page 177).

Chapter Twenty-five

Chocolate Orange Cake with a Twist

DIRECTIONS:

To begin, boil 12 cup filtered water in a microwave-safe cup or bowl. Once the water has reached a boil, carefully stir in the cocoa powder to create a thick chocolate pudding-like substance. Set aside to cool while you finish the remainder.

In a large mixing basin, combine all of the dry ingredients, including the chocolate chips, and stir to blend. After the batter is poured, this step keeps the chips from sinking to the bottom.

Then combine the eggs, butter, vanilla, and chia gel in a mixing bowl. As you can see in the photo, the mixture will be thick. After that, stir in the orange zest. Finally, stir the chocolate into the egg mixture (it's still hot, so be cautious not to touch it).

In a large mixing bowl, combine the wet and dry ingredients with a large wooden spoon. It will be a thick batter. Stir just until everything is combined, being careful not to over-mix.

In a greased cake pan, pour the batter. An 8 × 8 square pan, a 9-inch round pan, or a spring-form pan can all be used. Preheat oven to 350°F and bake for 30 minutes. A toothpick inserted in the centre should come out clean when done.

If you're going to serve this with mousse or whipped cream, make sure the cake is only warm, because any mousse placed on or next to it will melt. This cake's unusual flavour will leave an impression on your holiday guests! Ingredients (Dry)

7 tbsp cocoa powder (unsweetened)

34 cup of flour

1 cup packed brown sugar

12 teaspoon sodium chloride

12 tbsp baking soda

12 teaspoon powdered baking soda

1 pound chocolate chunks or chips

1 tablespoon orange zest, finely grated

Ingredients in liquid

2 eggs

12 cup water, filtered

5 tblsp. melted butter

5 tbsp chia seed gel

12 teaspoon vanilla extract

This orange sauce is convenient and delightful. You can thicken it to the consistency you want. It's shown here with the Sophisticated Chia Chocolate Orange Cake, but it may be used in any recipe. Serve with vanilla ice cream or with your favourite vanilla cake. What more uses do you have in mind for this orange sauce? This sauce is delicious hot or cold. It can be spooned over cake or ice cream or drizzled on a dish or bowl for a sophisticated look. This recipe yields around 3/4 cup orange sauce. The sauce will keep for approximately a week in an airtight container in the refrigerator.

Chapter Twenty-six

Orange Chocolate Sauce

DIRECTIONS:

All you need for this recipe is a stovetop pot. Over medium high heat, combine the sugar and cornstarch, then add the water and bring to a boil. The mixture should clarify up and thicken up. Return the liquid to a boil while whisking in the orange juice and concentrate. Reduce the heat to a low heat and add the butter. The sauce will thicken as it simmers longer, so cook until it reaches your preferred consistency. Finally, add the orange zest. 12 cup of sugar

14 cup filtered water 1 orange juice (about 12 cup)

cornstarch, 1 tablespoon

34 cup concentrated orange juice

1 teaspoon of butter

1 orange's zest

We think cupcakes are wonderful! They're the ideal portion control—somehow it's easier to eat one cupcake than it is to eat one piece of cake. Cupcakes that are light, sunny, and lemony will brighten your day. The cake is really delicate since we used cake flour instead of all-purpose flour. If you don't have cake flour, all-purpose flour can be substituted. (The gluten ratio is the crucial factor.) This recipe makes approximately ten big cupcakes.

Chapter Twenty-seven

Lemon Cupcakes

(Oh-So-Lemon)

DIRECTIONS:

Preheat oven to 375 degrees Fahrenheit. Using cooking spray, spray your muffin tin. There are 10 big cupcakes in this recipe.

In a mixing basin, sift together the flour, baking powder, and salt. With an electric mixer, whip the butter and sugar until light and fluffy in a separate bigger mixing dish. One at a time, beat in the eggs until each is fully absorbed. Combine the vanilla, chia gel, lemon juice, and 12 lemon zest in a mixing bowl. 34% of the flour mixture and 34% of the milk should be gently combined. Continue until all of the flour and milk has been combined. Do not overmix the ingredients. (No one enjoys a difficult cupcake!)

Fill the cups to about 34% capacity and bake for 17 minutes. (Check with a toothpick; these don't truly "brown.") Allow 10 minutes for the cupcakes to cool in the pan before transferring them to a cooling rack.

Once they've cooled, frost them with the "Not-so-Sweet Lemon Frosting," as shown.

12 cup flour for cake

2 tblsp. baking powder

salt to taste

sugar (cup)

2 lemons, grated (half the zest for the cupcake batter and half for the frosting)

Ingredients in liquid

6 tablespoons room temperature softened butter

2 tbsp chia seed gel

2 big room-temperature eggs

12 teaspoon extract de vanille

½ cup milk (low fat dairy or almond)

1 lemon juice teaspoon

We believe that smothering a delicious cupcake in fat and powdered sugar smothers the flavour. A light, not-too-sweet icing, on the other hand, provides a stunning presentation.

If you want to frost the cupcakes more than a few minutes before serving, keep them in the fridge with the whipped cream topping. On page 181, there are instructions. Because the bag of frosting keeps nicely in the fridge for a few days, we frequently frost cupcakes as needed immediately before serving.

Lemon Frosting That Isn't So Sweet

DIRECTIONS:

In a medium mixing bowl, beat the cream using an electric mixer. Beat the cream until it stiffens. Cream together the softened cream cheese. Repeat the process. The powdered sugar, lemon juice, and zest are then added. To incorporate, beat. The fun part of the frosting begins now. Fill a thick plastic bag halfway with the whipped cream mixture (such as a zip-top bag). Remove around 12" of the bag's corner tip. You now possess your own disposable pastry bag. Squeeze the whipped cream mixture into the bag's bottom and close it with a twist. Make a little swirl of frosting on each cup cake. 12 cup heavy cream

12 cup sugar powder

2 tablespoons low-fat cream cheese, softened

lemon juice, 1 teaspoon

1 teaspoon zest of lemon

Looking for a chocolaty, lighter version of banana bread? Try these lovely chocolate banana bars with swirls! This recipe is never heavy or dry, and it comes out more like a cake. You won't miss the fruity flavour combined with the wonderful cocoa swirl with three whole bananas within! The golden-brown swirled dessert will delight your visitors or family, and they won't believe how simple it was to prepare! This recipe makes one 13 x 9-inch pan of bars.

Chapter Twenty-eight

Swirl Bars with Chocolate Chia and Banana

DIRECTIONS:

To begin, cream the butter and sugar together until light and fluffy. Stir in the egg and vanilla essence until everything is well mixed. Combine the applesauce, gelled chia seeds, and mashed bananas in a mixing bowl. It makes no difference if a few little pieces remain. The finest flavour comes from ripe bananas with few spots. This mixture will be lumpy and yellowish at this point.

After that, combine the dry ingredients and stir well. Stir thoroughly as you gradually add the dry ingredients to the wet. All of the thick banana batter will now be in one basin. Scoop off roughly half of the batter and return it to the mixing bowl with the dry ingredients. To half of the batter, stir in 14 cup unsweetened cocoa until thoroughly incorporated. There may be banana chips visible, and the batter will be significantly thicker.

In a greased 13 x 9 baking pan, spread the non-chocolate half equally. Then, until all of the chocolate batter has been used, drop spoonfuls of it on top. Drag a knife through the chocolate batter to create a swirling pattern on the top of the dessert.

Preheat oven to 350°F and bake for 25 minutes. The edges should be golden brown when done, and a toothpick inserted in the centre should come out clean. You're ready to serve when you cut the cake into bars or squares.

These moist, delectable bars can be stored in an airtight container and do not require refrigeration.

Ingredients (Dry)

sugar (34 cup)

12 pound flour

1 teaspoon powdered baking soda

1 teaspoon bicarbonate of soda

12 teaspoon sodium chloride

14 cup cocoa powder

Ingredients in liquid

4 tbsp. melted butter

4 tablespoons chia seeds, gelled

1 egg

1 teaspoon vanilla extract

3 mashed bananas (approximately 112 cups)

12 cup applesauce, unsweetened

This is the lowest-fat, easiest, and most chocolaty cheesecake we've ever made! Expect something different than a classic, hefty cheesecake. Chia seeds were utilised to glue the crust and blend the contents together. This 8-inch cheesecake serves 12 people. You only need a small slice to "tame the chocolate beast," as the chia will make you feel satisfied.

Chapter Twenty-nine

Chia Cheesecake with Cocoa

DIRECTIONS:

Place a few graham crackers in the food processor and pulse until finely minced. Make your way to a measuring cup. Continue until you have 1 cup crushed grahams. Toss the graham crumbs with the chia gel and melted butter in a mixing basin. Press the crumbs into the bottom of the spring form pan once they've been wet.

Preheat the oven to 300 degrees Fahrenheit.

Remove the "dust" of cracker crumbs from the food processor. Combine the cottage cheese and two eggs in a mixing bowl. Blend until completely smooth.

Cream the cream cheese and sugar together in a large mixing dish with an electric mixer until creamy. Combine the cottage cheese, cocoa, flour, chia gel, and vanilla in a mixing bowl. Blend until smooth, then pour into the pie crust.

60–65 minutes in the oven Your magnificent cake's centre should appear to be set in the middle. Allow to cool for 20 minutes before loosening the edge of the cheesecake using a thin spatula or knife. Release the catch on the pan's side. Cool the cheesecake until it is just above room temperature, then wrap it in plastic wrap and chill for at least 4 hours. The crust's ingredients

1 cup chocolate graham crackers, finely crushed

2 tbsp chia seed gel

2 tablespoons butter, melted

The batter's ingredients

16 oz farmers cheese (low fat) (OR low fat Neufchatel OR cream cheese) 1 cup cottage cheese (low fat)

2 eggs

1 cup sugar (granulated)

12 cup cocoa powder, unsweetened

14 cup whole wheat flour

2 tbsp chia seed gel

1 teaspoon vanilla extract

To serve this cake to guests, we sprinkled it with powdered sugar and topped it with a dollop of low-fat sour cream. We topped the cake with puréed strawberries and a dollop of whipped cream the next day. Both were delicious.

Imagine the aroma of warm apple gingerbread straight from the oven. Your entire home will smell divine. This bread-cake is excellent because it is rich and dense despite the lack of shortening, oil, or butter. The peel of the grated apple is left on the bread for increased fibre, the chia boosts omega 3s, and with only a little sugar added, we'd think this cake is genuinely healthy. Apple gingerbread is simple to make with components you most likely already have on hand. The most difficult aspect is simply waiting for it to bake. This recipe makes one standard-size loaf (about 8.5 x 4.5 inches).

Chapter Thirty

Gingerbread with apples

DIRECTIONS:

Preheat the oven to 325 degrees and coat your loaf pan with cooking spray.

Except for the brown sugar, combine all dry ingredients in a mixing dish.

Combine the brown sugar, molasses, yoghurt, and eggs in a second, bigger mixing basin. Incorporate the eggs by beating or stirring them in. In a separate bowl, combine the dry ingredients. Next, shred the green apple that hasn't been peeled. In a large mixing bowl, combine the apple shreds and chia gel.

Preheat oven to 325°F and bake for 50–60 minutes. Check for doneness with a toothpick test.

Wrap foil around any leftover bread. When slightly warmed and topped with whipped, low-fat cream cheese, apple gingerbread is delicious in the morning. Ingredients (Dry)

1 cup flour (all-purpose)

12 cup oats (quick cooking)

12 tbsp baking soda

12 teaspoon powdered baking soda

cinnamon (2 teaspoons)

1 tsp ginger powder

nutmeg (1/4 teaspoon)

14 teaspoon cloves a pinch of salt

12 cup sugar (brown)

Ingredients in liquid

molasses (2 tablespoons)

2 tablespoons chia seeds, gelled

34% cup plain yoghurt

2 eggs

1 cup green apple shredded

Steven, one of our friends, was born with diabetes. We never know what to serve him for dessert besides a cup of sugar-free jell-o or a piece of fruit whenever he comes to dinner. We needed something unique that wouldn't affect his blood sugar levels. So this is our response to the problem. This sugar-free "cheesecake pudding" with strawberry or blueberry parfait looks festive, and it contains chia gel, which helps keep his blood sugar stable by preventing the conversion of carbohydrates to sugars. Although we are not fans of the sugar substitutes aspartame and acesulfame potassium, we believe that a little can't hurt. The size and height of your parfait glasses or dishes will determine how many servings you receive from this recipe.

DIRECTIONS: We've found that having all of the ingredients prepared and then constructing the parfait while making the coffee or tea after supper works wonderfully. The ginger snap cookies will absorb the moisture from the pudding if the parfaits are created too early.

Prepare the pudding according to the package guidelines for the "pie" form (not the pudding form). Whisk in the chia gel as indicated. Refrigerate after wrapping in plastic wrap. In a food processor, pulse the cookies until they are crumbs. Place the container in an airtight container.

Prepare and chill the fruit of your choosing.

Assemble right before serving by spooning alternate layers of pudding, crumbs, fruit chunks, and almonds. If you don't have parfait glasses, a stemmed wine glass would suffice. 1 sugar-free no-cook box

pudding with cheesecake (net wt 1 oz)

134 cup fat-free milk (use dairy because soy milk will not let the pudding set)

sugar-free ginger snap biscuits from the store, crushed fresh strawberries or blueberries

2 tablespoons choice of gelled chia nuts (if desired)

For breakfast, tea, or dessert, a light, fluffy, melt-in-your-mouth cake! This cake is so light that you may eat it at any time of day, but you'd better hurry because it'll be gone in no time! The top turns golden brown and crunchy, while the interior remains moist but not heavy. Fresh blueberries are ideal, although frozen blueberries would suffice. This recipe makes one 8 × 8-inch cake.

Chapter Thirty-one

Chia Blueberry Cake is light and fluffy

DIRECTIONS:

The eggs must first be separated. Whisk the egg whites in a separate bowl until stiff peaks form. After that, add 14 cup sugar and set away. Cream the butter with the remaining 34 cup sugar, salt, and vanilla in a separate dish. After that, add the egg yolks and chia gel. The finished product will be yellow.

Sift together the flour and baking powder, then gradually add it to the creamed mixture, along with the milk. After you've blended everything together, fold in the beaten egg whites. Fold in the egg white mixture gently until the batter is smooth and soft.

Prepare the berries: You don't want the whole cake to be covered in berries! Coating them in flour is a simple technique to prevent this. On a plate, sprinkle 2 tablespoons flour, then pour the berries on top. Roll them around in the coating until they're completely covered.

Fold in the coated blueberries carefully, then pour the batter into an oiled 8 × 8 pan. To serve, sprinkle with cinnamon and sugar to taste. About 1 teaspoon cinnamon and 2 teaspoons sugar are used. Preheat oven to 350°F and bake for 50 minutes. When done, a toothpick put into the centre will come out clean.

We don't think there will be much left over, but it can be saved in the refrigerator or even frozen and reheated for longer amounts of time. Of course, it tastes best when it's fresh!

Ingredients (Dry)

12 pound flour

14 teaspoon kosher salt

1 pound of sugar

1 teaspoon powdered baking soda

12 cup blueberries, fresh

2 tblsp flour (to coat)

blueberries

Ingredients in liquid

2 eggs (separated)

4 tbsp. melted butter (best if softened)

4 tbsp chia seed gel

1 teaspoon vanilla extract

¾ cup milk (low fat)

Topping:

to taste cinnamon and sugar

Chapter Thirty-two

Snacks and Appetizers

Looking for something to eat? Or something to stave off hunger till dinnertime? Try one of these chia appetisers or snacks. Instead of grabbing for a bag of chips or a candy bar in the afternoon, having a nutritious snack can make a significant impact in your health and energy levels. Chia provides you with sustained, non-jittery energy by adding protein and slowing the conversion of carbohydrates to glucose.

You can eat less by suppressing your hunger before a meal.

You'll be less inclined to overeat at meal time if you fill up on chia seeds before hand. Some of these appetisers may even be served as a meal. There's no regulation that says vegetables and dip can't be served as a meal. Why not if you or your family enjoy it and it is healthy?

Snacking on the wrong foods might ruin your healthy eating attempts.

When you're tired in the afternoon, a strong desire for a candy bar can arise. Without resorting to sweets, cookies, or chips, these foods will help you satisfy a nagging hunger or settle a sweet desire. You can get the instant crunch you want with a cracker or veggie stick dipped in garlic-y dip. With each chilly, refreshing bite, a chia popsicle can fulfil a sweet tooth with a rush of fruit flavour and wake you up. Cravings and fluctuating energy levels might be caused by blood sugar highs and lows throughout the day. Chia seeds contain two types of fibre that assist inhibit the conversion of carbs to glucose. This gives you a consistent, non-jittery supply of energy. When you take chia with a meal, the carbs are used more slowly. Chia also contains full protein, which is similar to that found in meat. (A rarity among plants!) The body must always use protein immediately away. It does not convert to fat or anything else; it simply delivers energy.

Chia aids in the transformation of beverages into food.

When chia seeds are gelled, they cause your digestive system to treat liquids as solids. To get to the liquid, the body must remove the soluble fibre off the outside of the seed shell. This allows the chia gel to linger in the stomach for longer, signalling that the stomach is still full. Because insoluble fibre (the coloured component of the seed shell) cannot be digested, it does not provide calories. It works as roughage, assisting food passage through the digestive tract.

In this approach, a chia drink, such as one of the many healthful green teas, might act as a snack. You'll never be bored with the variety of drinks, teas, and fruit juice options available. To regulate the fullness factor, use as much or as little chia as you prefer. Want to get rid of your hunger for good? 20 minutes before your meal, try a sugar-free chia drink. This allows the stomach's notoriously slow signalling system to begin transmitting fullness signals to the brain before the food is even served.

As an appetiser, crunchy toast slices and flavorful seasoned tomato make a winning combination. These delightful Italian-flavored slices can be eaten before or after a meal. When all of the plum tomatoes from the garden were ripe at the same time, Grandmother used to make a similar fresh tomato relish. This would be served as a side dish. We felt it was so wonderful that we would tweak very little and use it as a bruschetta topping. Depending on the size of your tomatoes, this should yield about one cup.

Chapter Thirty-three

Brochette with Plum Tomato and Chia

DIRECTIONS:

Combine all ingredients in a medium bowl and let aside for 10 minutes. This allows the flavours to blend and the sundried tomatoes to gradually rehydrate.

Brush the baguette slices with a little more olive oil and place them on a cookie sheet. This will keep the topping from soaking through the bread. Broil for 1 minute or more, or until the slices are lightly browned. Remove the cookie sheet from the oven and top the toast with the relish. Return to the oven for a minute to reheat the relish. Pay attention! Remove the cheese and sprinkle it on top. 3–4 chopped plum tomatoes (depending on size)

2 garlic cloves, minced

18 cup extra virgin olive oil

1 tablespoon chopped fresh basil leaves

1 tablespoon basil, dried

14 cup chopped sun-dried tomatoes

balsamic vinegar, 2 tablespoons

1 tablespoon chia seeds, dry

12 baguette, sliced diagonally

Topping with Romano/Parmesan cheese

If you're serving a large group, this recipe can simply be doubled.

This should be your go-to pesto recipe in a pinch. It takes only a few minutes to make in your food processor and is quite flexible and tasty. Serve it over tortellini or turkey burgers, or even chicken breasts. This delicious pesto is created with fresh spinach and basil. It has a vivid green colour, is delicious, and tastes quite fresh. The spinach and fresh basil are high in vitamin A, while the olive oil aids digestion and vitamin and mineral absorption. The chia helps to combine all of the flavours and gives the pesto more substance. This recipe yields half a cup of pesto.

Chapter Thirty-four

Chia Pesto with Spinach

DIRECTIONS:

Place the spinach, basil, and garlic in a small food processor fitted with the chopping blade attachment and pulse until smooth. Chop. Process the olive oil, parmesan, broth, and chia seeds until they make a thick, fragrant paste. 1 cup spinach leaves, fresh

14 cup basil leaves (fresh or dried)

2 teaspoons grated parmesan

12 tablespoons extra virgin olive oil

1 garlic clove, chopped

14 cup chicken broth (low salt)

1 teaspoon chia seeds, dried

We enjoy this pesto on a burger with a piece of mozzarella cheese!

This no-cook cranberry pomegranate spread is delicious, versatile, and easy to make! Serve it with crackers, chips, cheeses, or on a sandwich to impress your guests and family! This quick, healthful blend requires no cooking; simply whip out the food processor. Everything about it is packed with health advantages. It's bright and cheery, and it'll wow you with its incredible flavour. To share, make one small bowl of relish.

Chapter Thirty-five

Panini and Canberry Pomegranate Zippy Chia Relish

DIRECTIONS:

In a colander, rinse the cranberries. Remove any berries that are underripe or overripe. Rinse and shake the cilantro to dry it. Remove the cilantro's long stems with kitchen scissors. Remove the seeds from the pepper and discard them.

In a food processor, combine the cranberries, cilantro, onion, and pepper. To finely chop, pulse a few times. After that, stir in the lime juice, agave nectar (or stevia), dry chia, and pomegranate arils. To combine everything, pulse twice quickly. 12 oz. fresh or frozen bag

cranberries

1 handful cilantro, chopped

pepper, jalapeno

de-seeded

lime juice, 3 teaspoons

14 cup arils de pomegranate

14 cup agave nectar OR sugar substitute

selection (such as stevia)

14-inch red onion circular

1 teaspoon chia seeds, dried

It is critical not to over-chop, as this will result in slush. It should be a thick, spreadable slurry. To use with crackers, cheese, or chips, simply spoon the relish into a colourful dish and serve. Microwave the chicken breast thoroughly before making the panini. After that, slice thinly and set away. If you want, you may cook the chicken on your counter-top grill. If you like, you can use deli sliced provolone cheese.

Spread the mixture on top of your favourite bread slice. Place the chicken breast slices on top. If desired, top with a thin deli slice of provolone cheese and the last bread slice. Spray your skillet (or panini machine) with cooking oil spray, as well as the outside of the bread, to keep it from sticking. Place the sandwich on a grill or in a skillet over high heat for about 2 minutes, or until toasted and the cheese has melted. On page 198, the paninis are shown with rustic whole-grain cranberry bread.

Some traditional black bean dips can be a touch calorie and flavour heavy. When serving vegetables and crackers, the dip can sometimes mask the flavours of the vegetables. This black bean dip is modest, but it packs a punch. Simply pull out your food processor and make up a batch in no time. You don't want to ruin your good intentions by providing extra vegetables with a bad dip. Every item in this recipe is healthy and delicious! This silky dip goes great with veggies, chips, and more. This recipe serves one medium bowl of dip.

Chapter Thirty-six

Dip of light black beans

DIRECTIONS:

In a food processor, combine all of the ingredients except the chia and hot sauce. Purée until the mixture is smooth. Add the chia seeds and a pinch of cayenne pepper. Adjust the amount of hot sauce to your preference. Please remember that flavours develop over time. If you're going to keep the dip in the fridge until needed, make the last modifications right before serving so it doesn't get too heated. 12 can black beans, washed

12 cup cottage cheese (low-fat)

3 tablespoons chopped white onion

1 celery stalk, sliced into bits

12 inch chunk of deseeded jalapeo pepper

1 or 2 garlic cloves

12 teaspoon cumin powder

1 teaspoon coriander powder

1 teaspoon chia seeds, dry

1–3 dashes spicy sauce (if you dare)

This simple microwave dip can be prepared ahead of time and simply reheated when your guests arrive. If you know you'll be busy after the party starts, this is a terrific option. It's also excellent for leftovers. You're halfway there if you can open a frozen carton of chopped spinach. This is a hearty and thick dip. This recipe serves one medium bowl of dip.

Chapter Thirty-seven

Warm Spinach and Chicken Dip

DIRECTIONS:

If you're using rotisserie chicken from the store, shred roughly one cup. If using an uncooked chicken breast, chop it into large bits and set it in a baking dish with a low side.

Cover and microwave on high for 2 minutes, then flip and rotate the pieces. Cook for another minute or two until no pink remains. You can begin shredding after the mixture has cooled slightly. 1 frozen 10-ounce package

spinach, chopped

roughly 1 shredded chicken breast

onion, 2 tablespoons

cream cheese, 3 oz.

12 cup Swiss cheese, shredded

2 tbsp plain yoghurt

2 tbsp chia seed gel

nutmeg (14 teaspoons)

1 de-seeded and diced tiny sweet red pepper

1 teaspoon crushed red pepper

Place the frozen spinach brick in a covered dish and microwave according to package instructions. Cook the spinach and wring off the excess water with a fork. Combine the chicken, onion, cream cheese, Swiss cheese, yoghurt, chia gel, red pepper flakes, and nutmeg in the same casserole dish. Stir everything together. Warm the dip on half power for 2–3 minutes. This dip can also be kept in the refrigerator until needed for your celebration.

Hummus is a spicy and nutritious Mediterranean dish. This bean and spice mixture is delicious as a dip, spread, or topping. If you've discovered how delicious hummus is, you've undoubtedly also learned how costly it is! A little plastic tub of store-bought hummus can cost up to $6. Even for one person, the small tubs don't last long because it tastes so good. Making your own hummus is a great way to cut costs. This will yield roughly a cup of hummus.

Easy Chia Lemon Hummus DIRECTIONS: This can be made in minutes if you have a food processor, micro chopper, or even a blender. To begin, puree the chickpeas until completely smooth. Then puree all of the remaining ingredients until smooth. Your hummus is now ready to spread over pitas, tortillas, crackers, as a veggie or chip dip, or even to substitute mayonnaise in sandwiches. It doesn't get any simpler than that! 1 can garbanzo beans or chickpeas

(drain and rinse)

2 garlic cloves

lemon juice, 2 tablespoons

2 tablespoons extra virgin olive oil

1 teaspoon zest of lemon

2 tablespoons chia seeds, gelled

a quarter teaspoon of chilli powder

What are the health benefits of this hummus recipe? Chickpeas or garbanzo beans are used in all hummus recipes. Beans are high in plant protein and fibre in general. Garbanzo beans are no exception, and they contain several important amino acids as well. These are nutrients that your body requires but cannot produce on its own. (You'll find tyrosine, tryptophan, and phenylalanine, to name a few.) Chickpeas are slow to digest due to their protein and fibre content. Hummus has a low glycemic index, which means it won't spike blood sugar levels. This helps you maintain a constant level of energy. Lemon juice contains vitamin C, but did you know that it also contains the trace minerals copper, manganese, molybdenum, and iron? Each of those minerals, in trace levels, can aid you with everything from sulfite detoxification to heart health.

These small pieces will give you a nice fibre boost while also satisfying your chocolate appetite! These aren't brownies, and they're not meant to be eaten in large slices—just a small bite as an afternoon snack or an after-dinner treat would suffice. They have a fruity, chocolaty, and mocha flavour. This filling, chewy snack could possibly be a preventative precaution for you. However, keep in mind that this dish contains sugar, so don't overdo it. This recipe makes one 8 × 8 snack pan.

Chapter Thirty-eight

Fruits and Chia

Nibbles of Chocolate Prunes

DIRECTIONS:

Preheat the oven to 350 degrees Fahrenheit and spray an 8 × 8 square baking dish with cooking spray.

Combine 7–8 prunes and 2 tablespoons boiling water in a small chopper, food processor, or blender. Chop till completely smooth. If necessary, add 12 teaspoon of water at a time. The paste will be quite thick.

Melt the chocolate squares in the microwave for around 40 seconds.

Place the melted chocolate, prune purée, eggs, sugar, and vanilla in a mixing dish. Blend until smooth. Add the chia gel and mix well. Combine the flour, salt, instant coffee, and baking powder in a large mixing bowl. Stir everything together. 4 oz. unsweetened chocolate squares a quarter cup of prune purée

12 cup of flour

sugar (34 cup)

2 eggs

2 tbsp chia seed gel 1 teaspoon powdered baking soda salt to taste

1 tablespoon instant coffee OR instant espresso coffee

1 teaspoon vanilla extract

Spread into the baking pan that has been prepared. Bake for 30 minutes, or until a toothpick inserted in the centre comes out clean.

Allow it cool completely before cutting into bite-size squares.

Bone Health and Dried Plums? Studies on how to preserve strong bones throughout life have recently been conducted. In many investigations, one fruit stands out above the rest: the dried plum. Dried plums appear to contain particular polyphenols that inhibit the breakdown of bone, allowing new bone to develop. "Over my career, I have examined various fruits, and none of them come close to having the effect on bone density that the dried plum does," says Dr. Bahram Arjmandi. Dr. Bahram Arjmandi is the dean of research at

Florida State University and the director of the Center for Advancing Exercise and Nutrition Research on Aging (FSU). 1

As a healthy snack, how about a popsicle? Definitely, especially when they're prepared with fruit like these! Popsicles are a great snack since you can make them all in under ten minutes and then take one out of the freezer whenever you want something sweet. The banana fudge pop is so nutritious that it may be eaten for breakfast.

The banana is responsible for the texture and flavour of these pops. When frozen, a banana does not turn into an icy mess like most fruits do. It has a softer, creamier texture that is more attractive. When you add a little banana in with your favourite fruits, it keeps them from turning frosty while without giving the whole dish a banana flavour.

These popsicles are made entirely of fruit and include no added sugar. Popsicles are colourful, enjoyable to eat, and appealing to children. Why not try a chia pop after school instead of a bag of chips? The chia seeds in this recipe help you stay full until your next meal. The size of your moulds will determine how many popsicles you receive from each recipe.

Popsicle with Chia Watermelon Slices

These are adorable and entertaining! Making each pop look like a slice of watermelon is straightforward. If you wish to make a dessert version, replace the "watermelon seeds" with small chocolate chips. Did you know that kiwi seeds are beneficial to your health? Make sure to just remove the rough core of the kiwi and not the small black seeds.

Peel and core the kiwi, then blend the banana and kiwi together in a food processor until smooth. To determine how tart the kiwi is, taste the combination. Kiwis are grown all year in many countries, and some are sweeter than others. To sweeten, add the 14 teaspoon stevia and stir one more. For the watermelon part:

12 bananas, medium 1 cup chunks of watermelon

1 teaspoon chia seeds, dried

For the section of green "rind":

14 or 12 medium bananas

1 kiwi

14 teaspoon stevia extract (if desired)

Fill the moulds with the kiwi mixture for the remaining 14 minutes, then insert your popsicle handles and freeze.

The kiwi is an extremely nutritious fruit! It has more vitamin C than an orange, the same amount of potassium as a banana, and plenty of fibre! Alpha-linolenic acid, as well as vitamins C and E, are found in kiwi seeds.

No one will believe how healthy this popsicle is since it is so delicious. It has the appearance and texture of a fudge bar, but it only contains four components, each of which is beneficial to your health. Use cocoa that is pure, raw, unsweetened, and not Dutch-processed. It has the highest antioxidants and flavonols, which are beneficial to your health. You won't need any additional sweeteners because the banana is so high in natural fruit sugars.

Banana Chocolate Fudgies

DIRECTIONS:

In a food processor, blender, or micro chopper, puree the ingredients until smooth. Fill your popsicle moulds with the mixture, then freeze. 1 large banana (ideal if bright yellow and without spots)

112 tablespoons chocolate powder, unsweetened

1 teaspoon chia seeds, dry

3–4 tablespoons rice OR almond milk, unsweetened

If you want to spice things up, try making a peanut butter version: 1 tablespoon unsweetened natural peanut butter and 1 tablespoon more milk of your choice

Raspberries are a refreshingly sweet and tangy summer delicacy. They're also available as a frozen fruit, which is less pricey. Frozen raspberries are a healthy, vibrant, and eye-opening addition to these pops. The watermelon helps to keep these from being overly sour. The half-banana gives it a subtle creaminess without making it taste like a banana pop.

Watermelon Raspberry Popsicle

DIRECTIONS:

In a food processor, blender, or micro chopper, puree the ingredients until smooth. Fill your popsicle moulds with the mixture, then freeze. 12 bananas, standard size (yellow, without spots works best)

14 cup raspberries, frozen

34 cup chunks of watermelon

1 teaspoon chia seeds, dry

Chapter Thirty-nine

Chia Beverages

By just adding chia gel and stirring it around, you can turn practically anything into a chia beverage. You don't have to worry about the acidity of orange juice preventing the chia from gelling because it has previously gelled in water. Chia seeds can be used to fruit juices, smoothies, shakes, teas, sports drinks, and just about anything else! However, you should be aware that it will remove the fizz from carbonated beverages.

You won't run out of tastes to try thanks to the wide variety of unsweetened teas available. Some of the fruited teas don't even taste like tea, so if you don't like tea, try varieties like natural raspberry or natural blueberry. These flavours are also appealing to children. Want to give your tea a boost of flavour? 1 teaspoon concentrated frozen fruit juice

Do you like a sweeter tea? Take stevia or xylitol into consideration. They're natural sweeteners made from plants (stevia is a leaf, xylitol is a bark) that the body doesn't recognise as sugars. They have a light sweetness to them. Artificial sweeteners, such as aspartame, have been shown to enhance hunger in certain people. They can also induce allergic responses or adverse effects. Stevia is a low-cost sweetener that can be found in most supermarkets. Just a smidgeon will suffice! Sweetening beverages organically with stevia or agave nectar (or even honey) may entice children away from high fructose corn syrup soft drinks.

You can brew tea by the cup or make a pitcher at night and keep it in the fridge for whenever you need it. Preparing simple snacks or drinks ahead of time cuts down on subsequent excuses.

Chia is also great in drink mixes or fast powdered drink mixes (often known as "to-go packages") that are supposed to be used with a water bottle. Simply flavour as directed on the packet, then add your chia seeds, gelled or dry. To blend, give the bottle a good shake, and you're ready to go.

Fresca Chia

It all started with a drink! On hot summer days, the ancient Mexican natives produced this delicious drink. Cold water, sugar cane juice, lime, and chia were used. They stayed hydrated thanks to the vitamins in lime juice and the nutrients in chia seeds. The soluble fibre on the outside of the chia seed helps to moisten the colon by being eliminated by the intestines. You may enjoy this old delight with this simple recipe! 1 cup of iced water

lime juice, 2 tablespoons

1 tbsp chia seed gel

to taste stevia

Chia fresca makes one serving.

DIRECTIONS:

Simply combine all ingredients in a glass and serve immediately, with ice cubes if desired.

Mint, Lemon, and Chia Seed Green Tea

Do you really want to get rid of hunger? Take this tea! Green tea polyphenols increase leptin, the hunger-suppressing hormone. Mint is also a natural appetite suppressor, so when combined with chia, it's a formidable force against hunger. According to a recent study, persons who drink minted green tea (approximately 2—3 cups per day) consumed 2,800 calories fewer per week than those who did not drink any tea. (And that wasn't even include the chia!) Fresh mint should be added for the greatest flavour. 4 tea bags (green)

½ a lemon's juice

1 tablespoon (or more) chia gel

2–3 leaves of mint per serving

Approximately 2 pints

DIRECTIONS:

After the tea has steeped, remove the tea bags. Cool the tea, then add the chia gel and lemon juice once it has to room temperature. Sweeten to taste with stevia or a natural sweetener of your choice. Add 2–3 mint leaves per cup when ready to serve. Eat the leaves as well for the optimum results.

For the chia enthusiast, chia concentrate beverages are filled with health and nutrients. They do not, however, have the consistency of a typical drink. The chia seeds are equally distributed throughout the beverage, giving it a thicker texture and a stronger fruit flavour. Bottles of chia drinks like this can be seen in trendy supermarkets. Did you know you can make your own for a fraction of the price at home?

This short shot of chia concentrate is made with this little recipe.

Beverages with Chia Concentrate

DIRECTIONS:

To blend and melt the concentrate, stir everything together. Make sure you're using 100% fruit juice concentrate, as some frozen or bottled juices may contain high fructose corn syrup, colours, or artificial flavourings. You don't want to undo all your hard work! 1 tablespoon juice concentrate of your choice

3 tblsp. of water

3 tbsp chia seed gel

Chia Teas with Fruit

Simply brew the tea according to package recommendations, cool, and whisk in your chia gel and stevia to get the fruited chia teas shown here (peach and raspberry).

Chia Seed Beverages

Chia seeds can also be used in hot beverages. A teaspoon or tablespoon of already gelled chia will do the trick nicely. For a cappuccino flavour, the coffee is served with hot frothed almond milk.